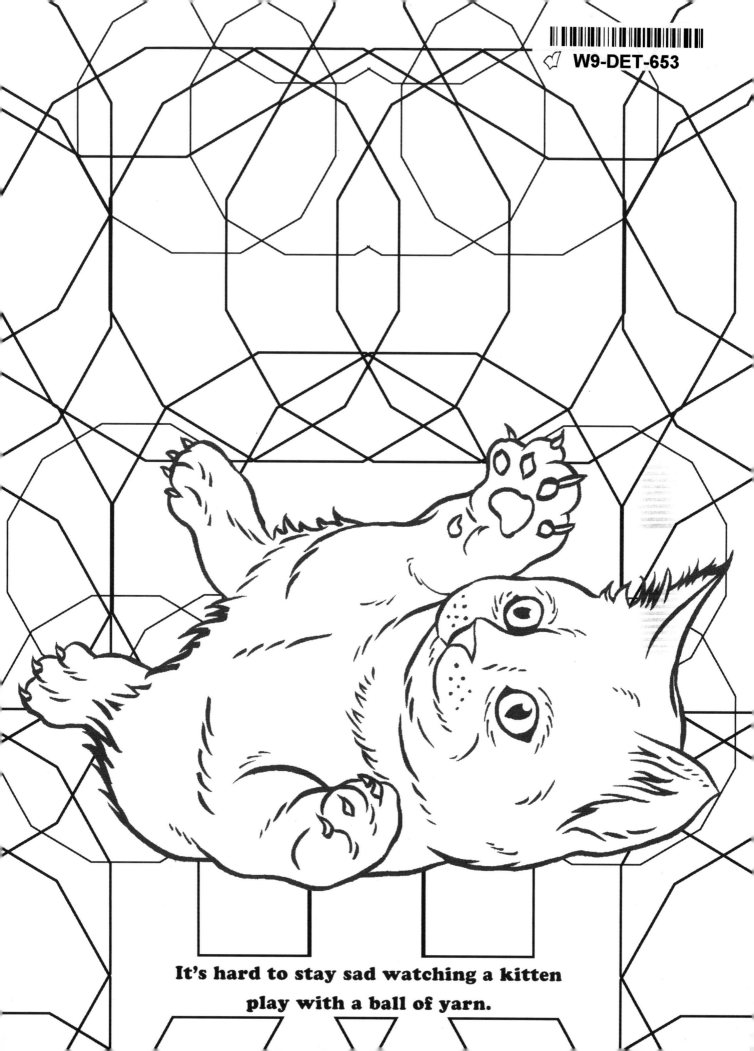

It's hard to stay sad watching a kitten play with a ball of yarn.

W9-DET-653

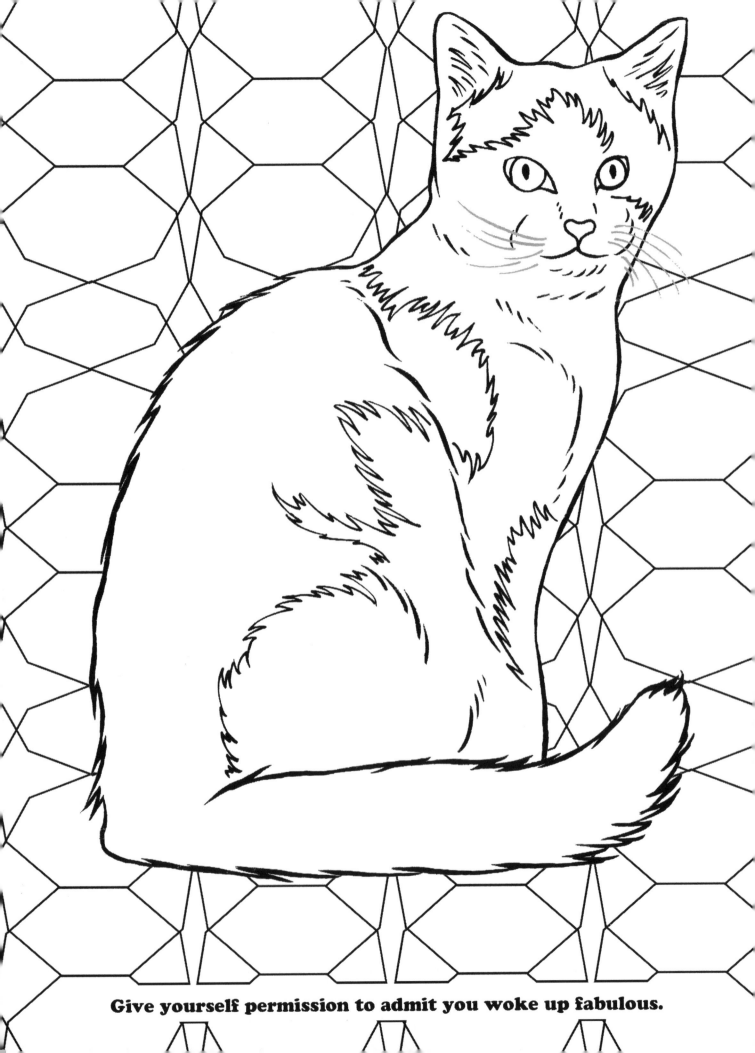

Give yourself permission to admit you woke up fabulous.

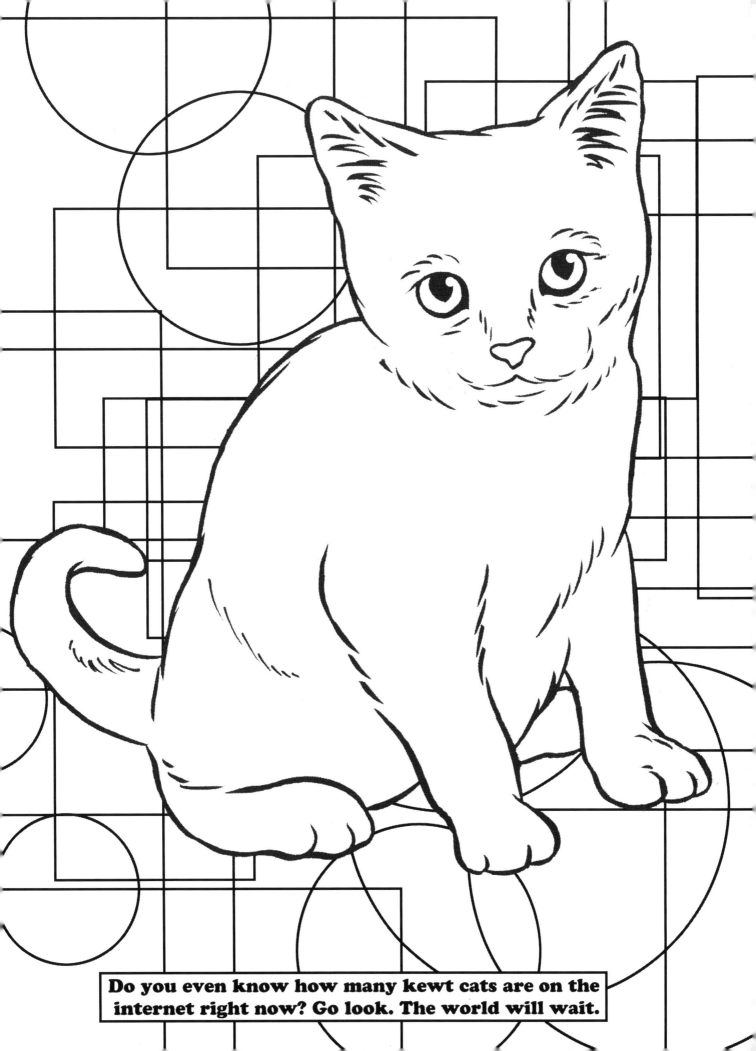

Do you even know how many kewt cats are on the internet right now? Go look. The world will wait.

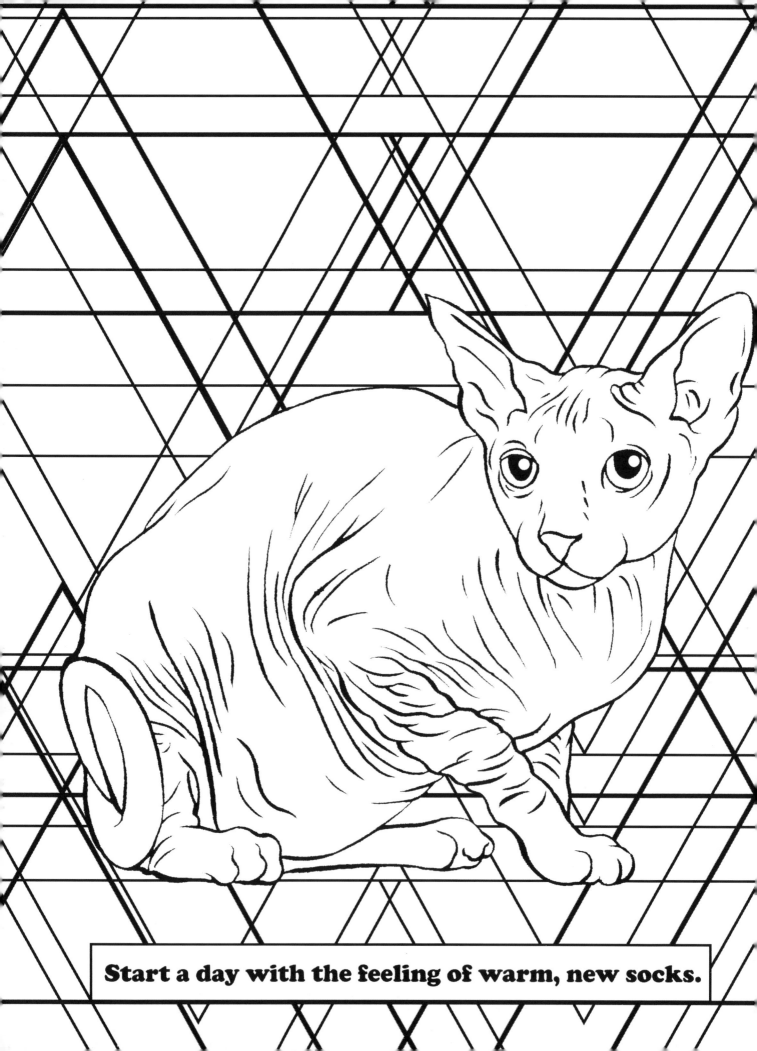

Start a day with the feeling of warm, new socks.

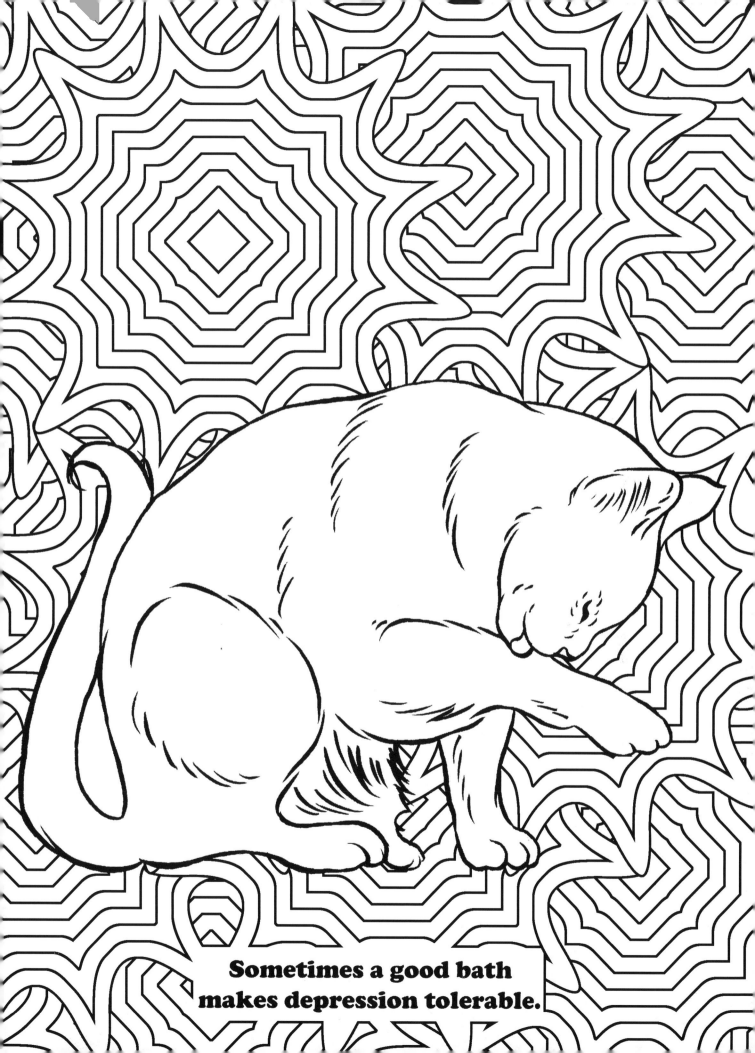

Sometimes a good bath
makes depression tolerable.

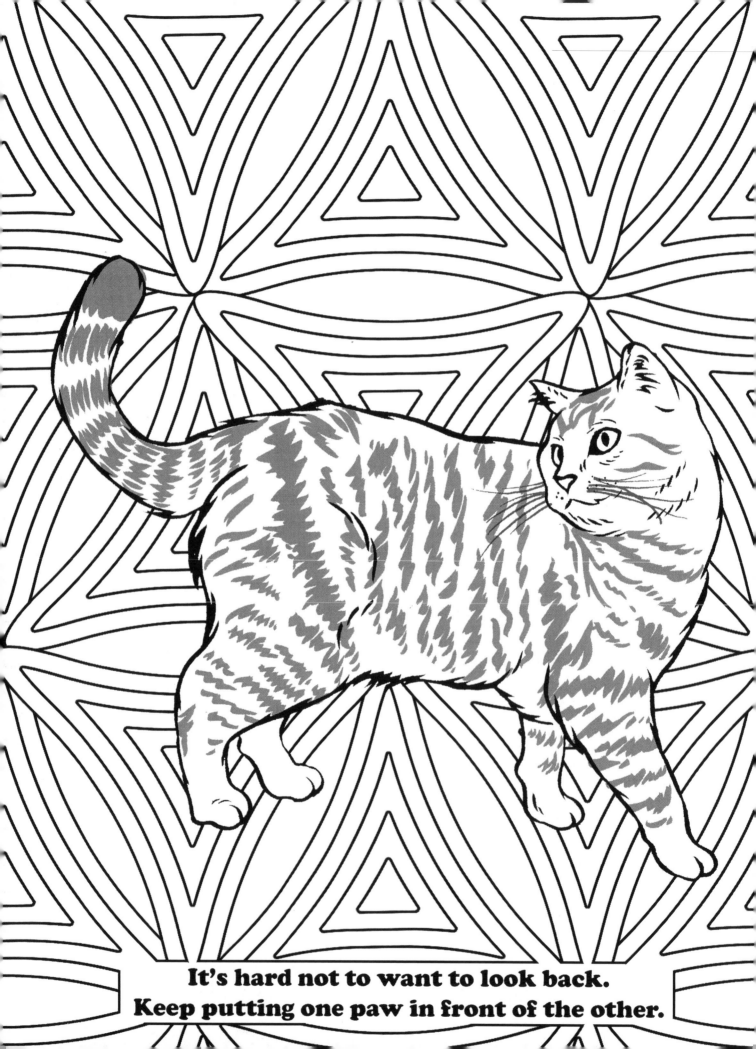

It's hard not to want to look back.
Keep putting one paw in front of the other.

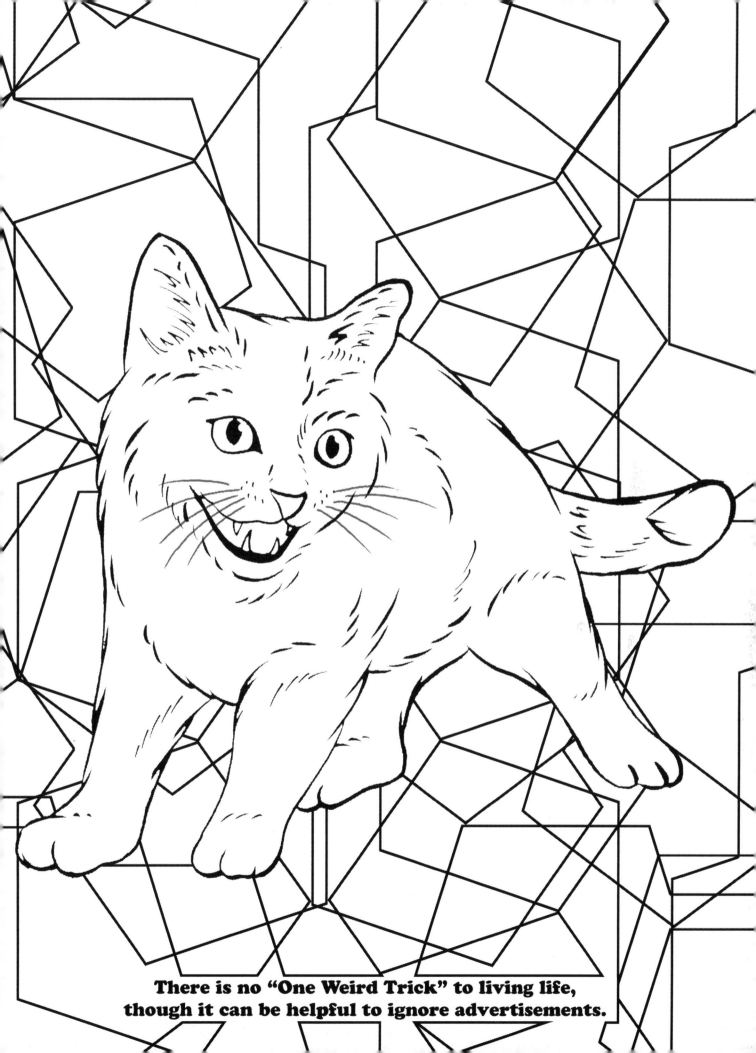

There is no "One Weird Trick" to living life,
though it can be helpful to ignore advertisements.

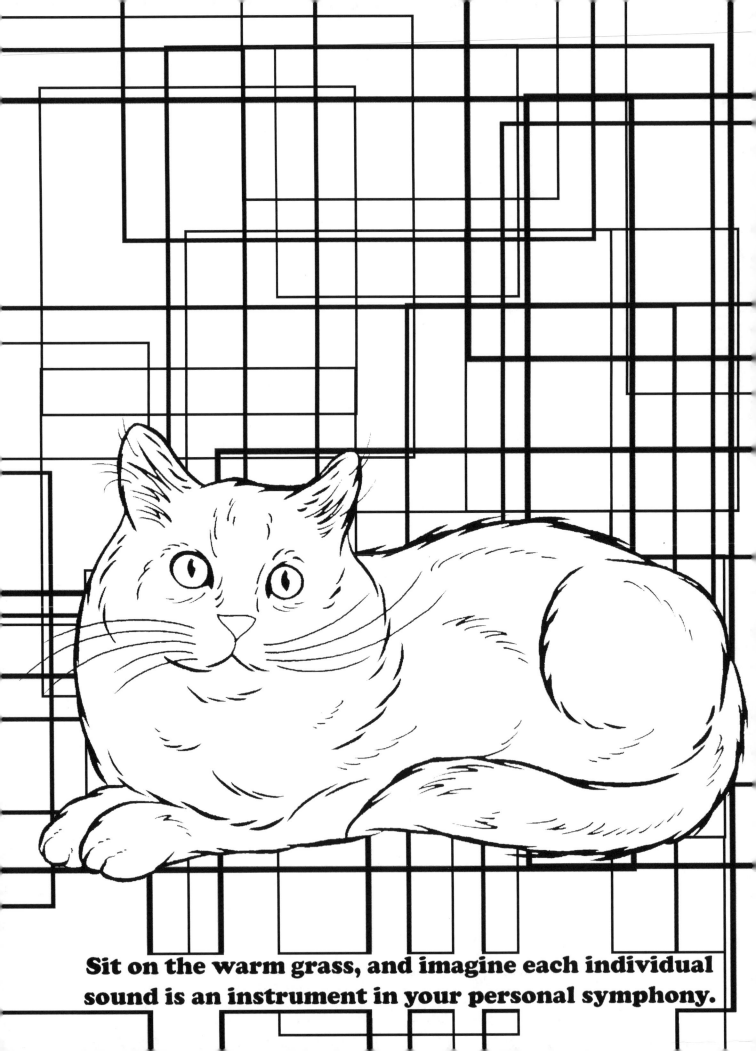

Sit on the warm grass, and imagine each individual
sound is an instrument in your personal symphony.

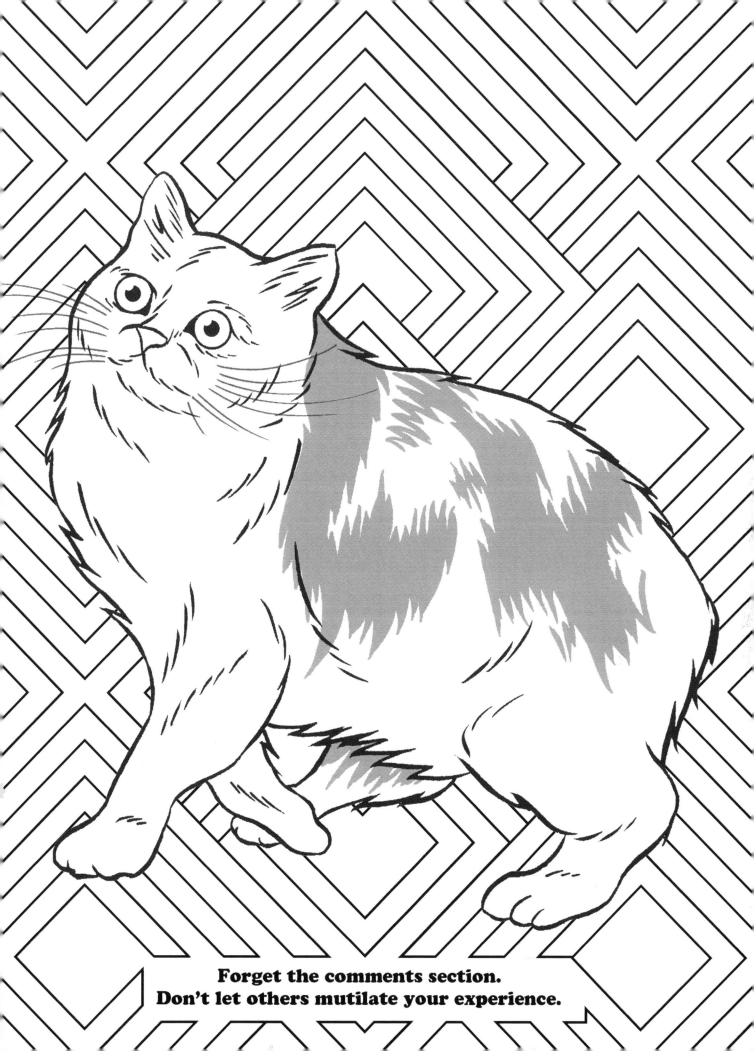

Forget the comments section.
Don't let others mutilate your experience.

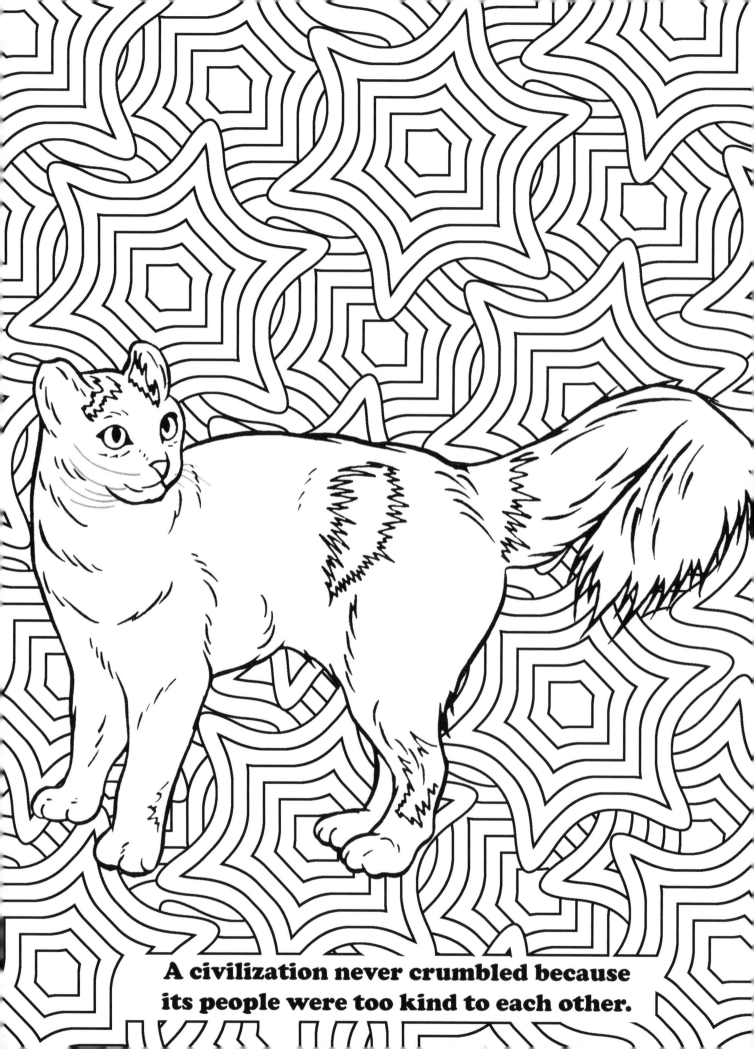

A civilization never crumbled because its people were too kind to each other.

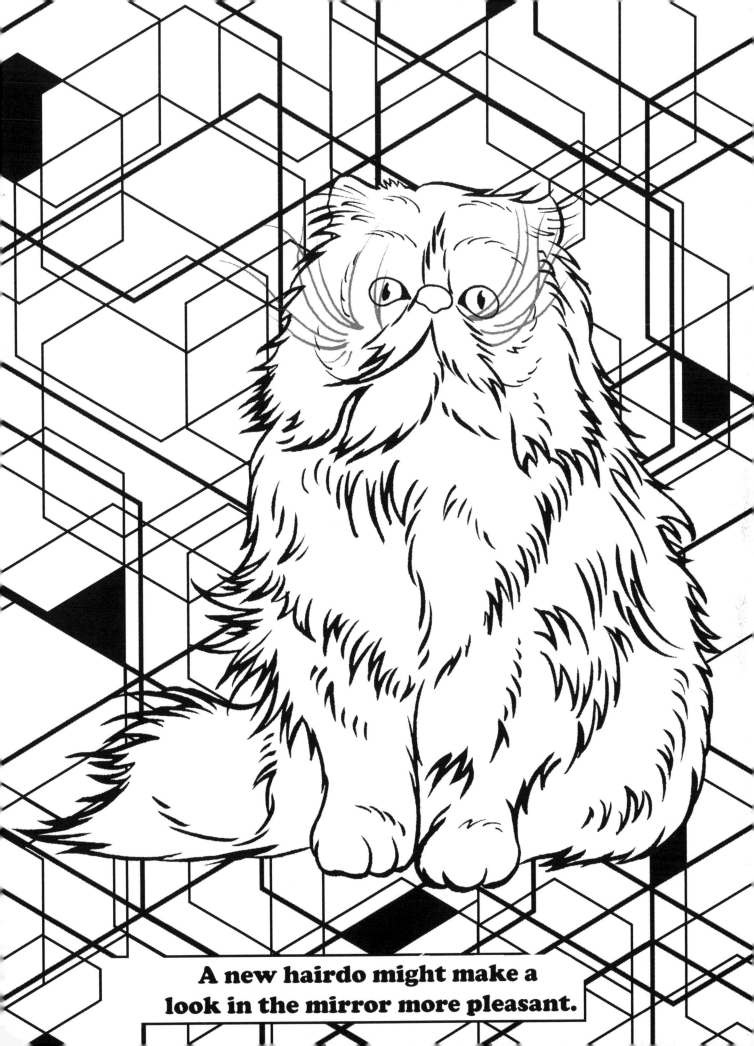

A new hairdo might make a look in the mirror more pleasant.

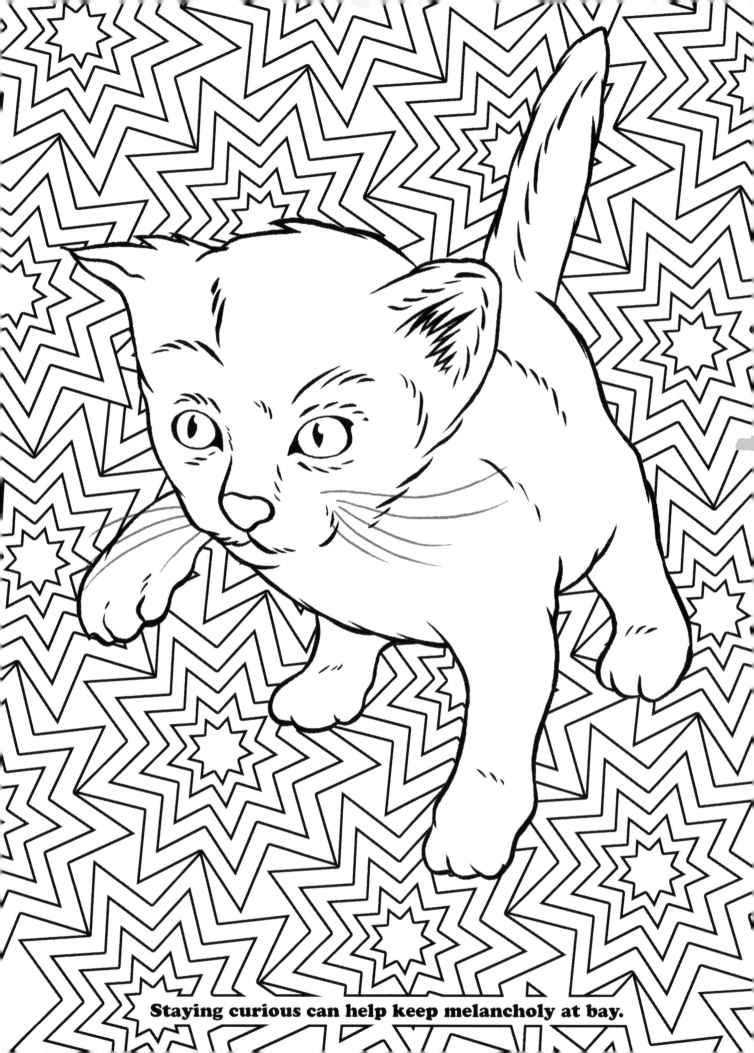

Staying curious can help keep melancholy at bay.

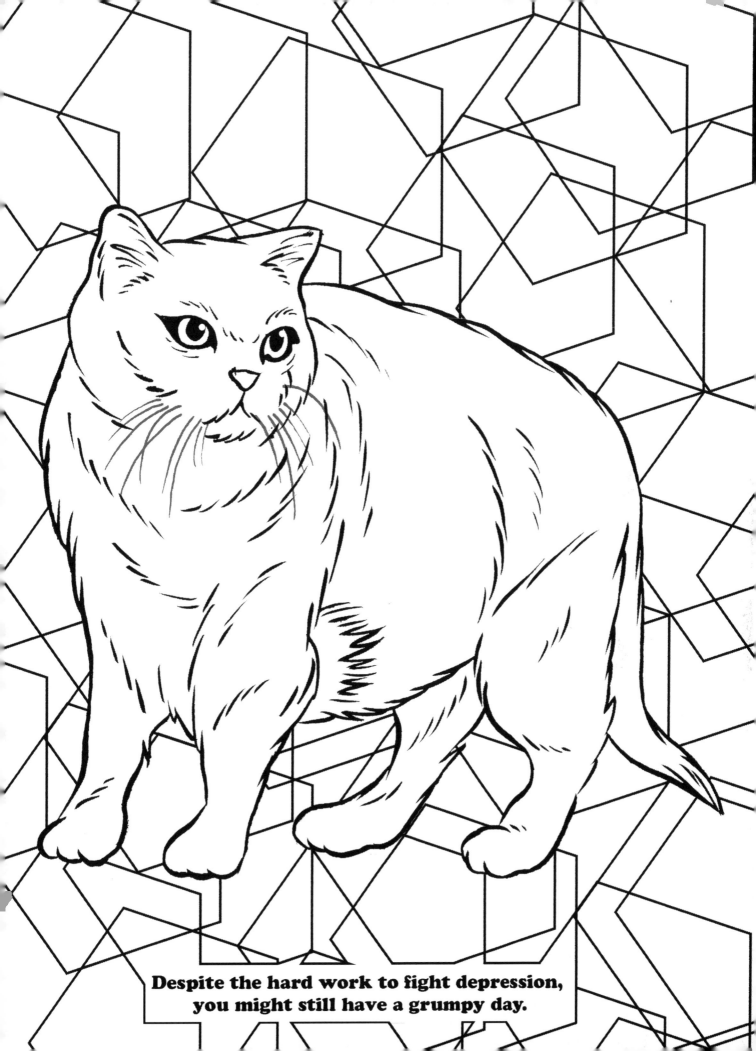

Despite the hard work to fight depression,
you might still have a grumpy day.

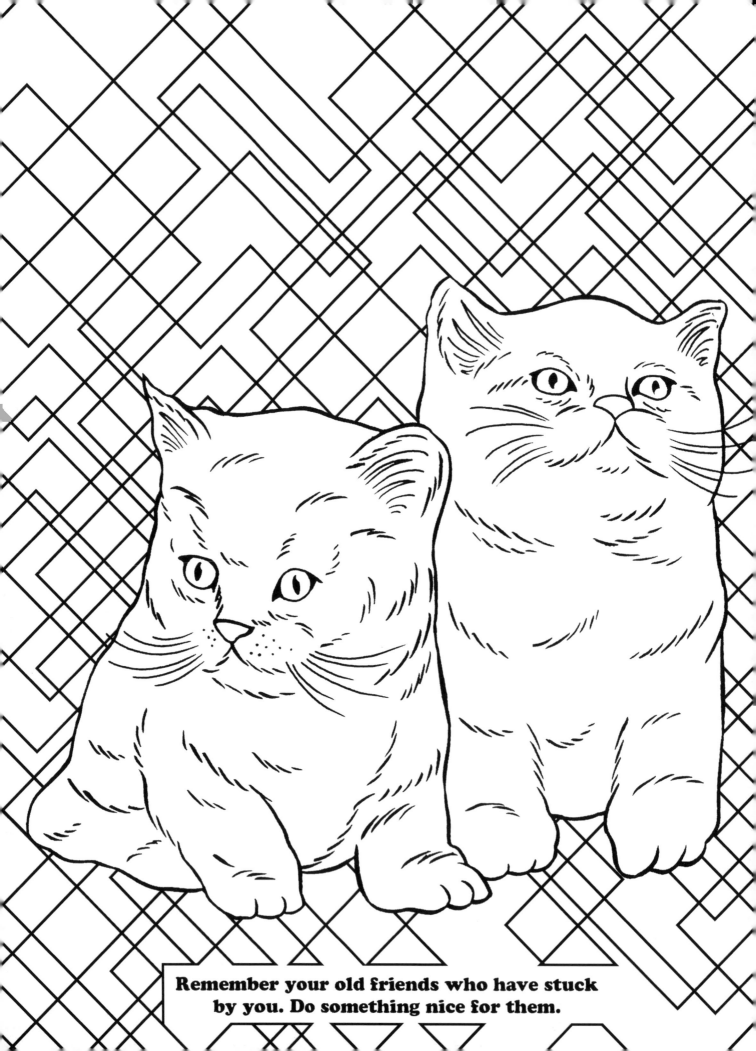

Remember your old friends who have stuck
by you. Do something nice for them.

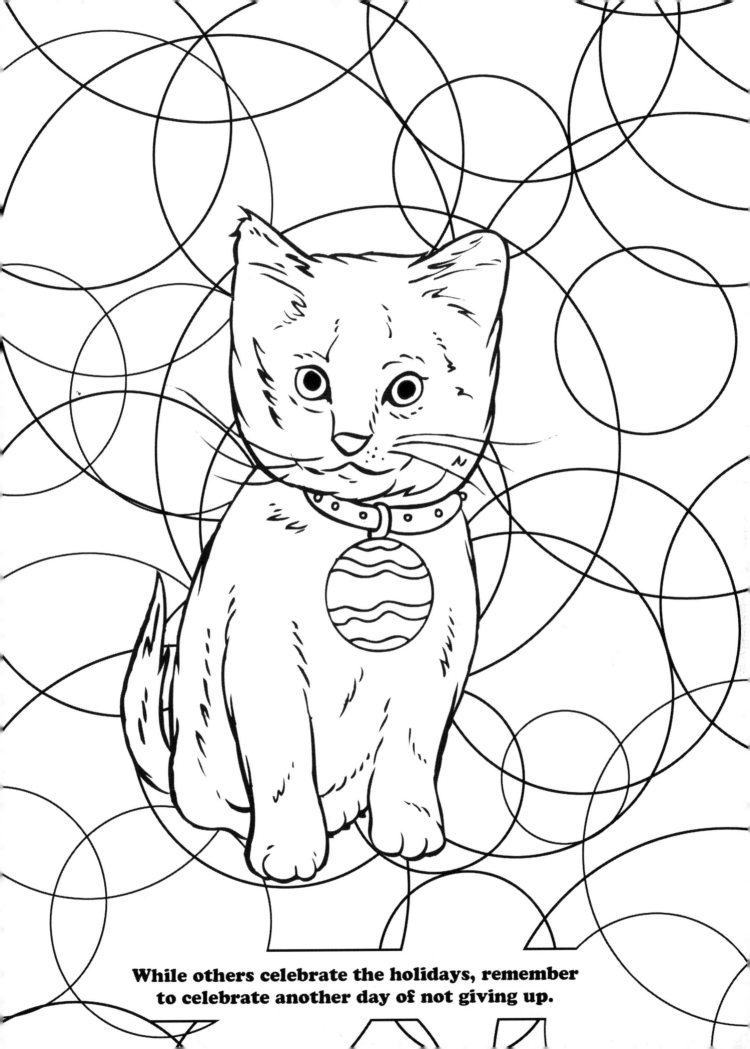

**While others celebrate the holidays, remember
to celebrate another day of not giving up.**

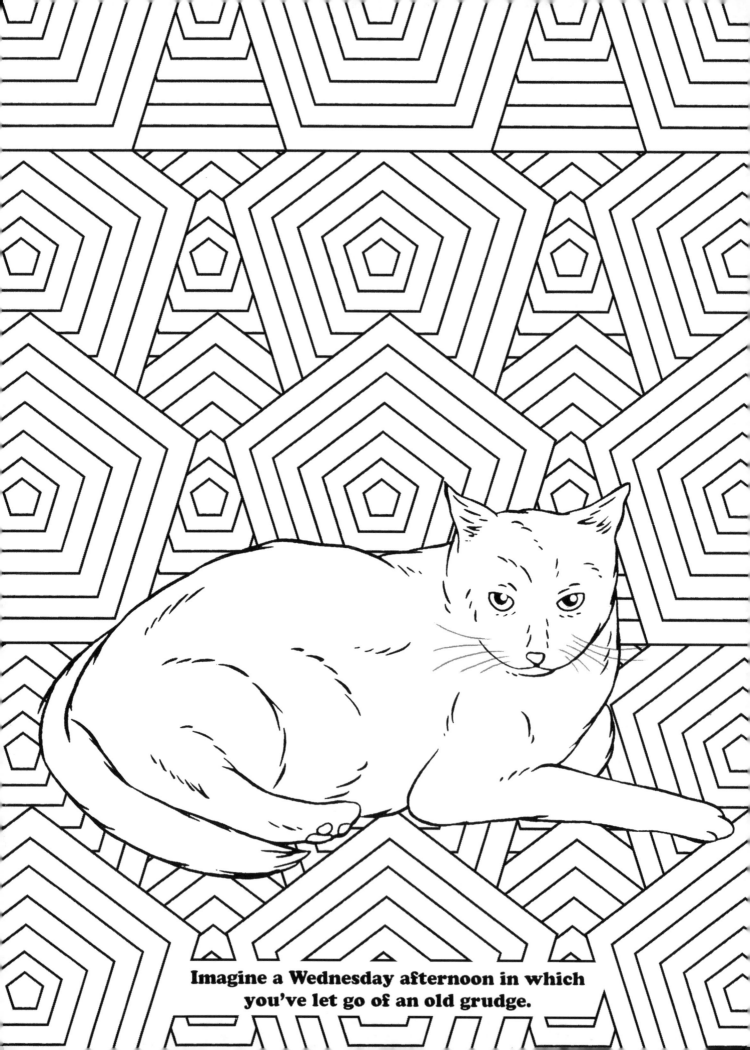

Imagine a Wednesday afternoon in which
you've let go of an old grudge.

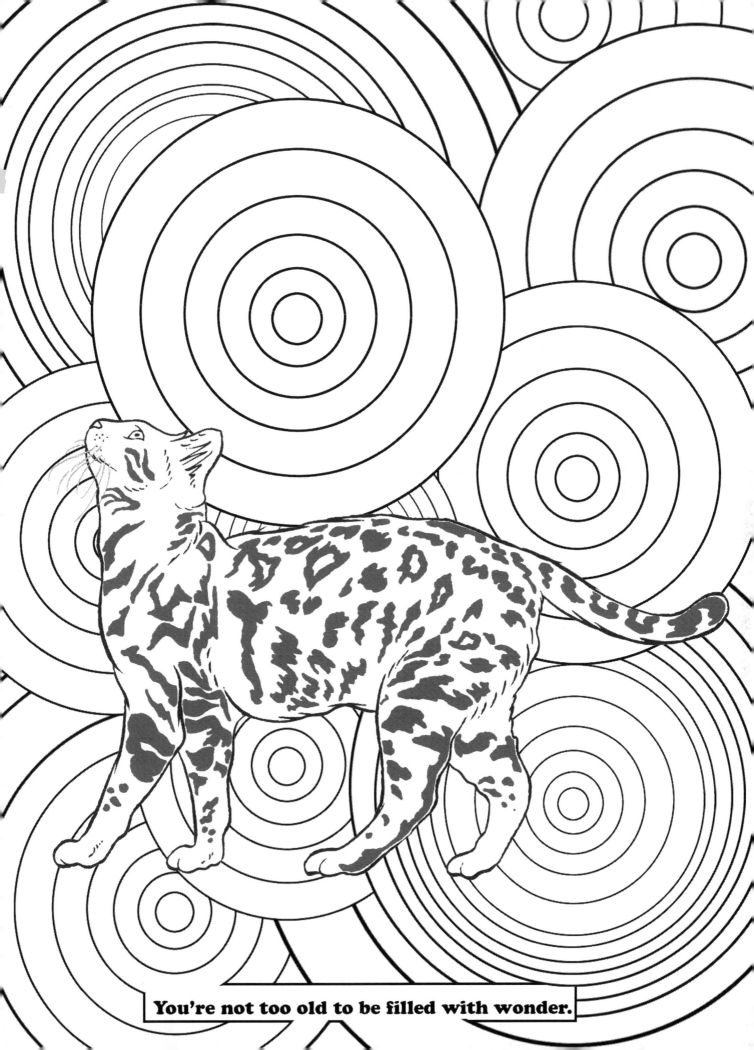

You're not too old to be filled with wonder.

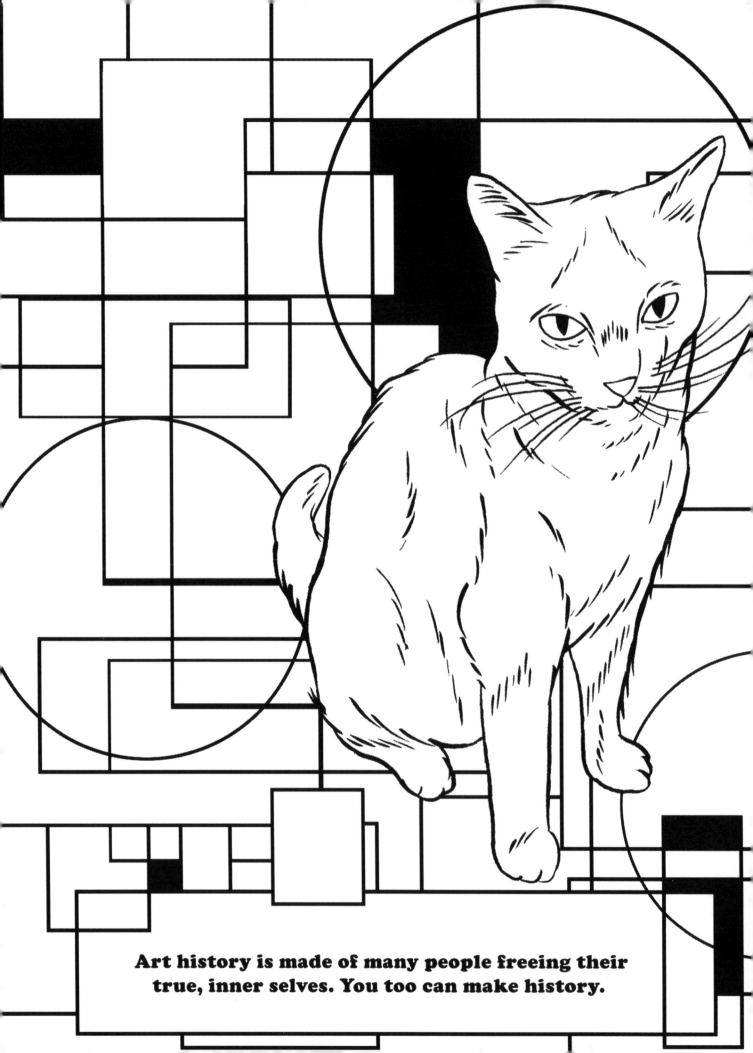

Art history is made of many people freeing their true, inner selves. You too can make history.

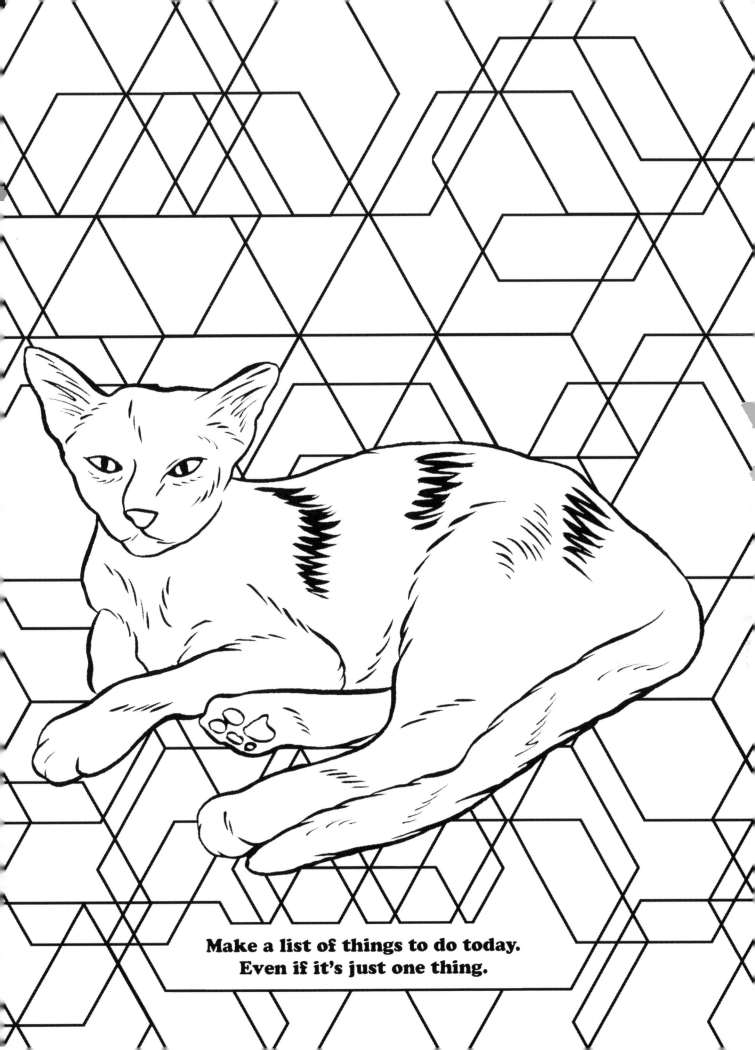

**Make a list of things to do today.
Even if it's just one thing.**

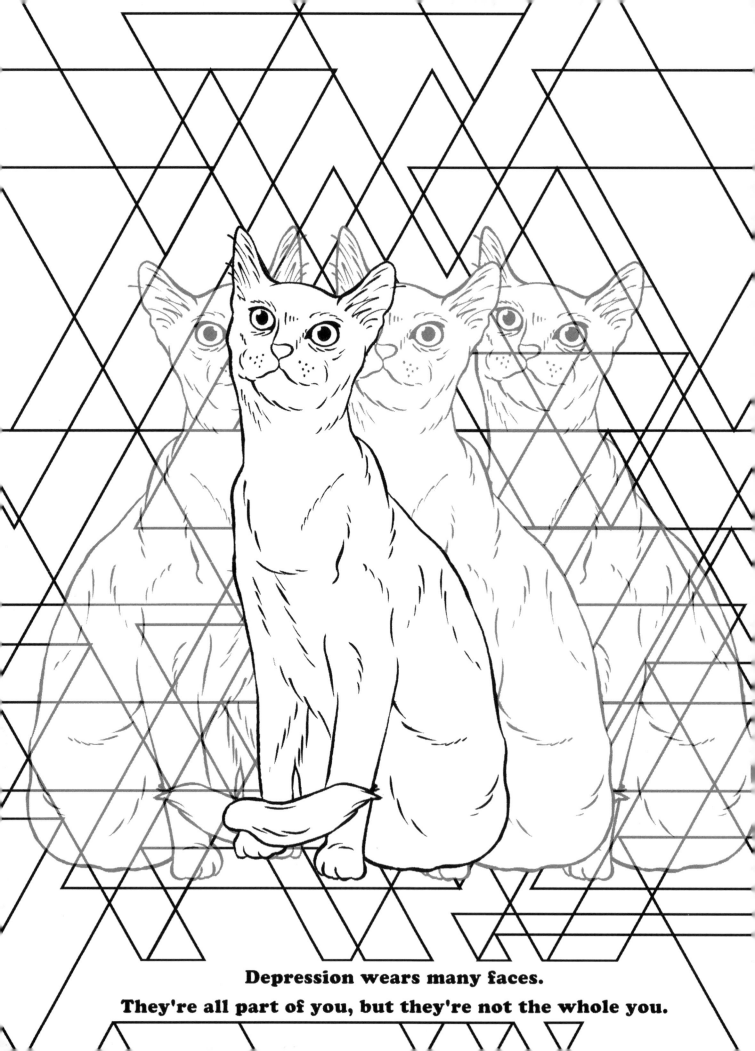

Depression wears many faces.

They're all part of you, but they're not the whole you.

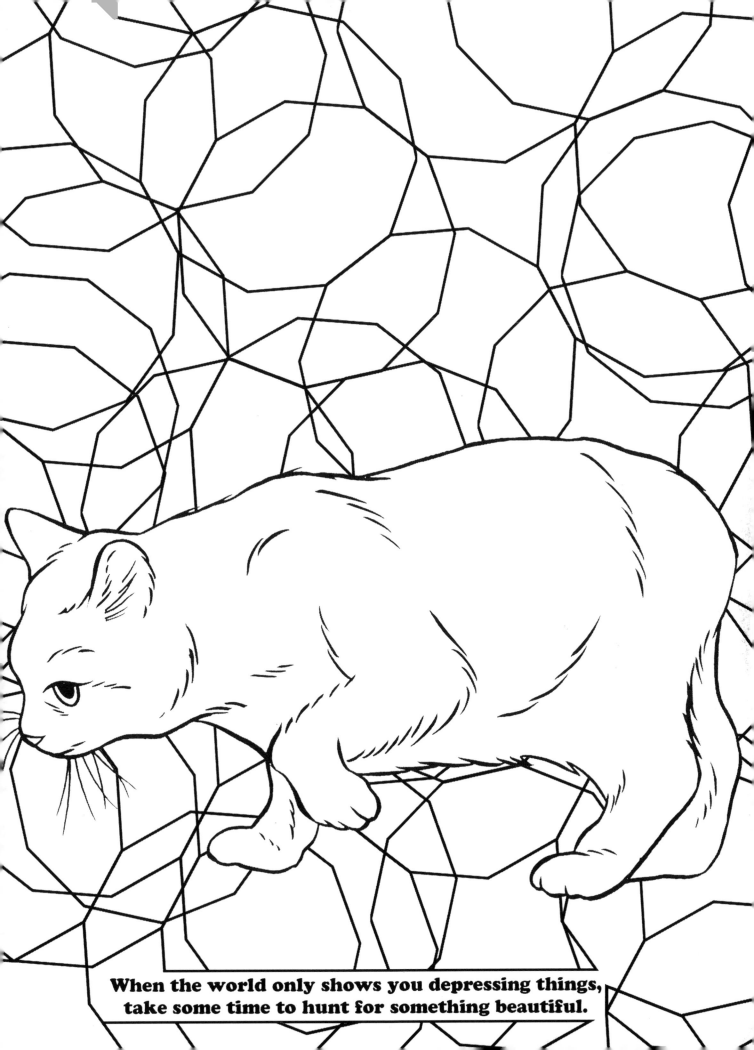

When the world only shows you depressing things, take some time to hunt for something beautiful.

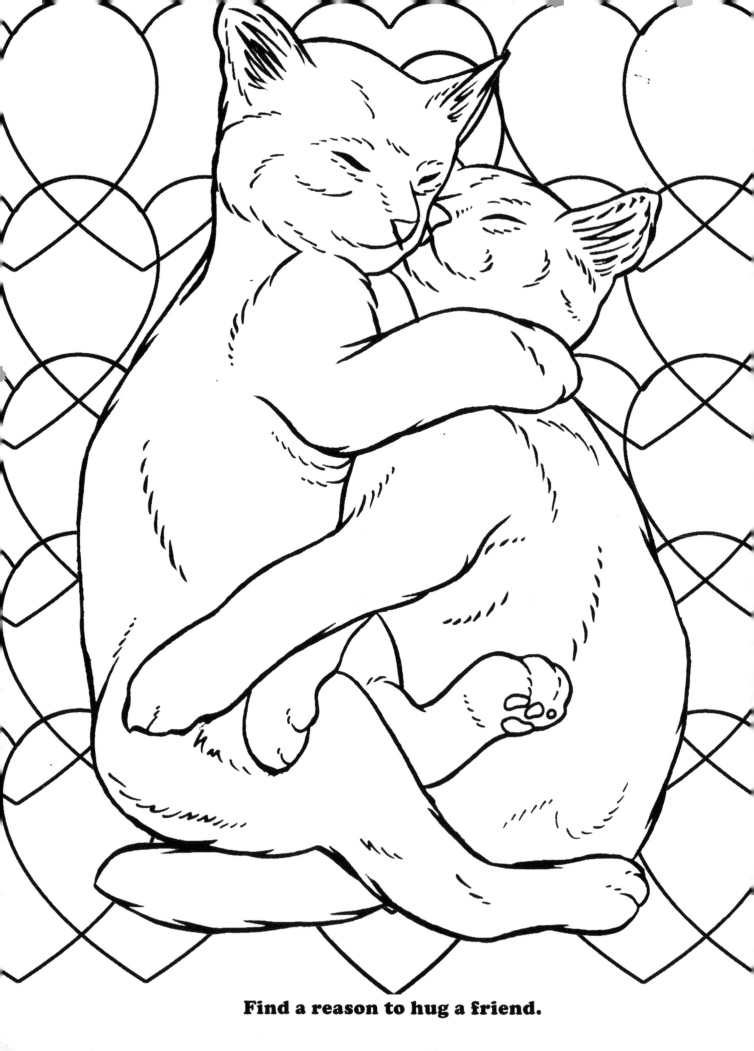

Find a reason to hug a friend.

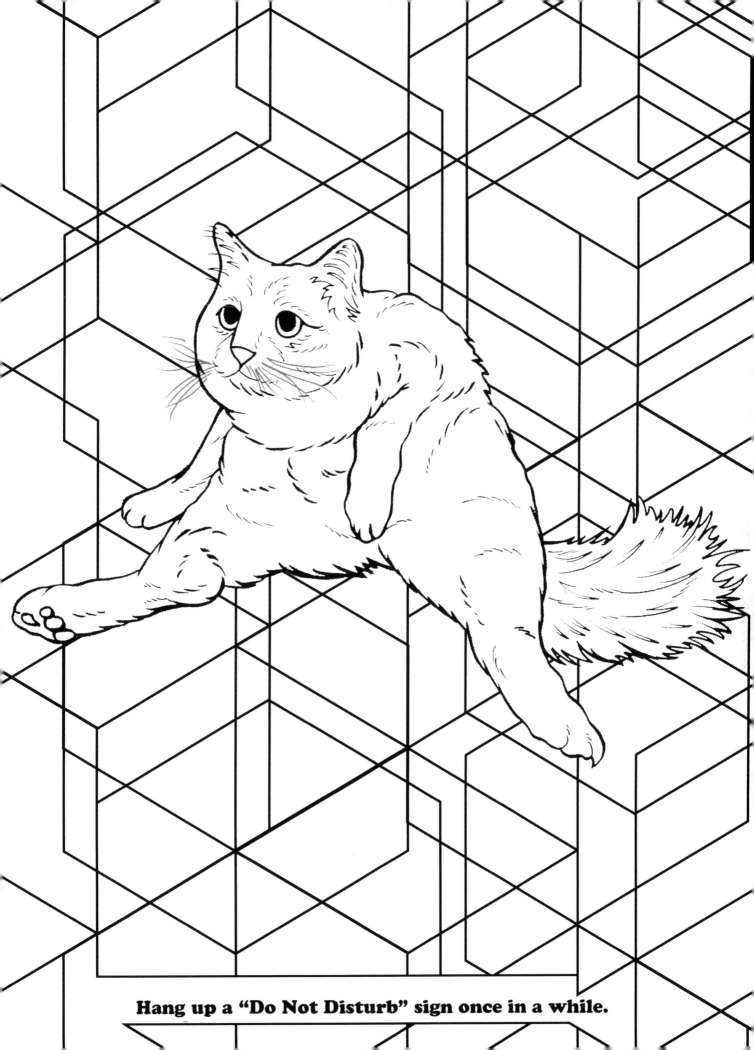

Hang up a "Do Not Disturb" sign once in a while.

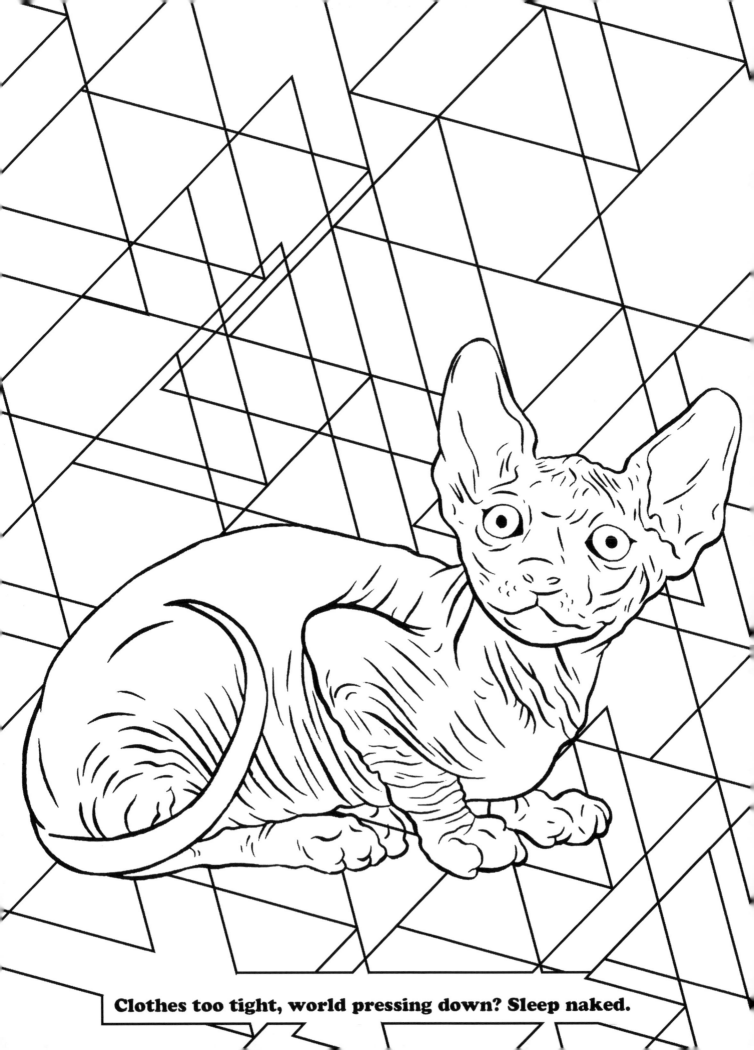

Clothes too tight, world pressing down? Sleep naked.

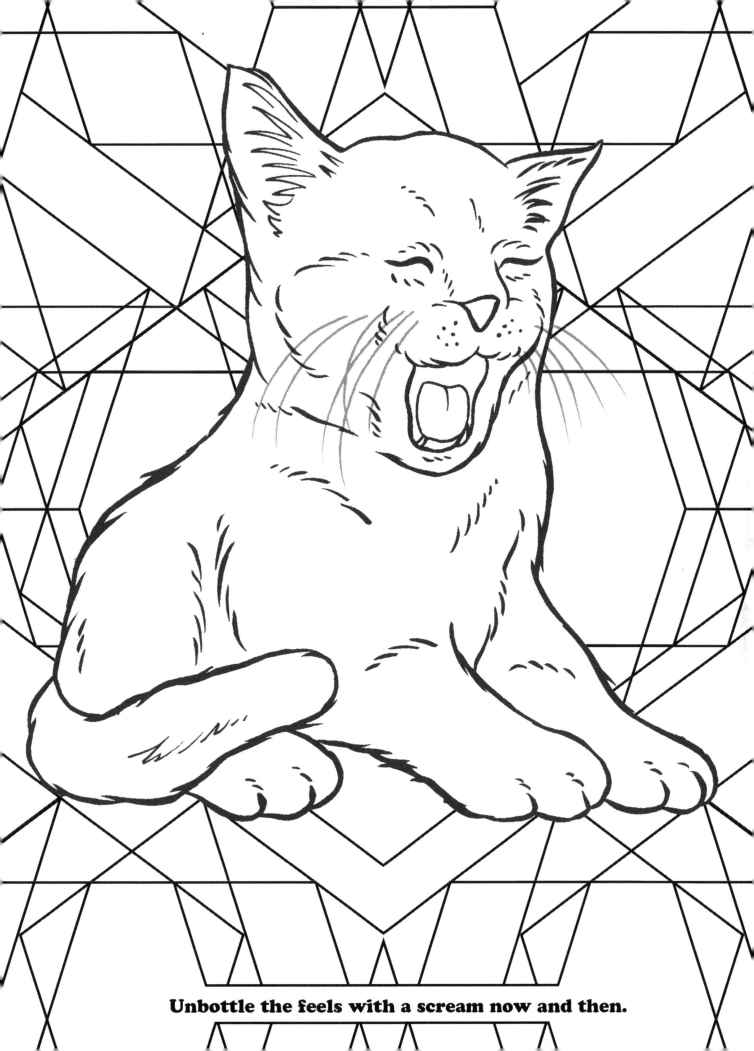

Unbottle the feels with a scream now and then.

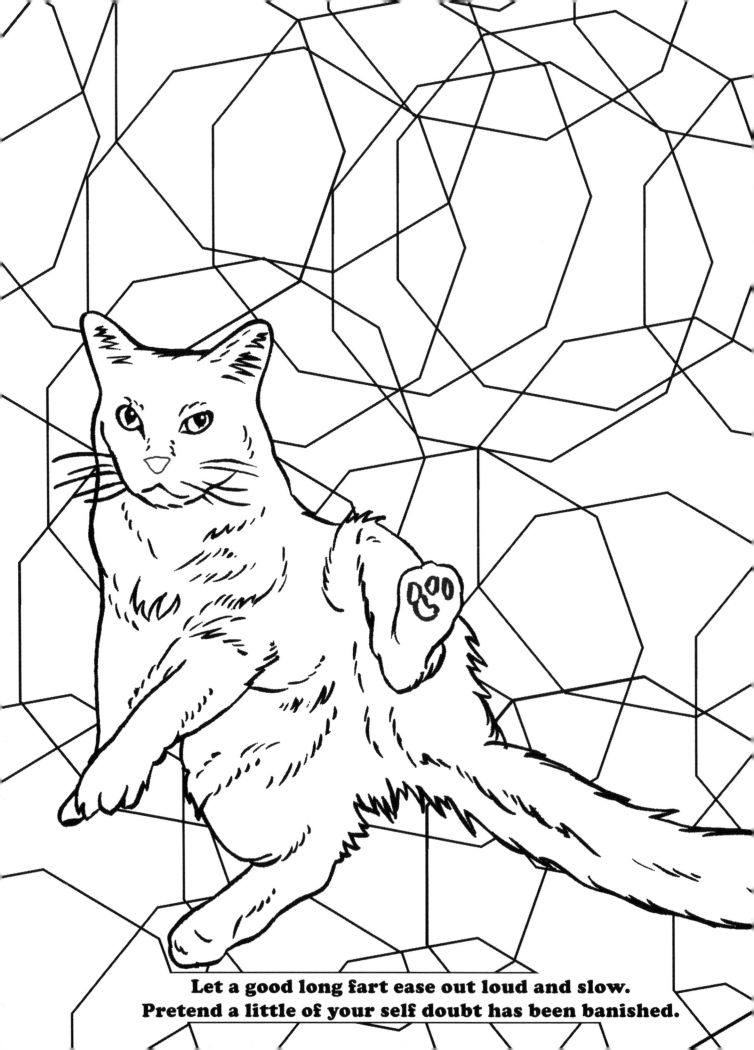

Let a good long fart ease out loud and slow.
Pretend a little of your self doubt has been banished.

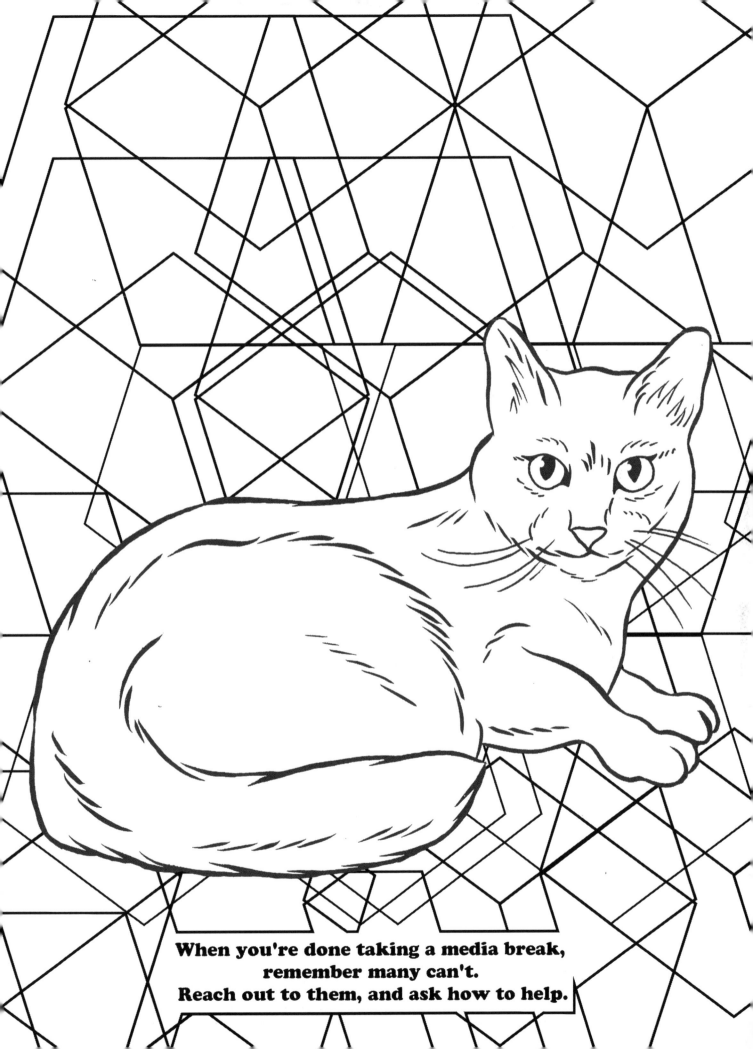

When you're done taking a media break,
remember many can't.
Reach out to them, and ask how to help.

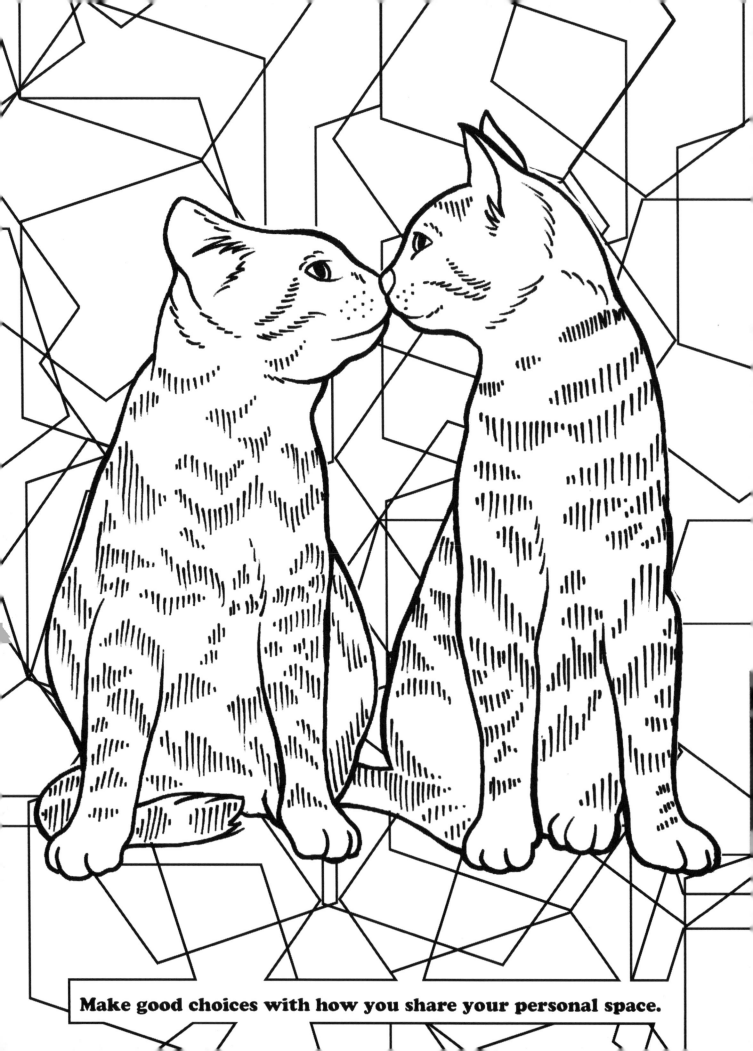

Make good choices with how you share your personal space.

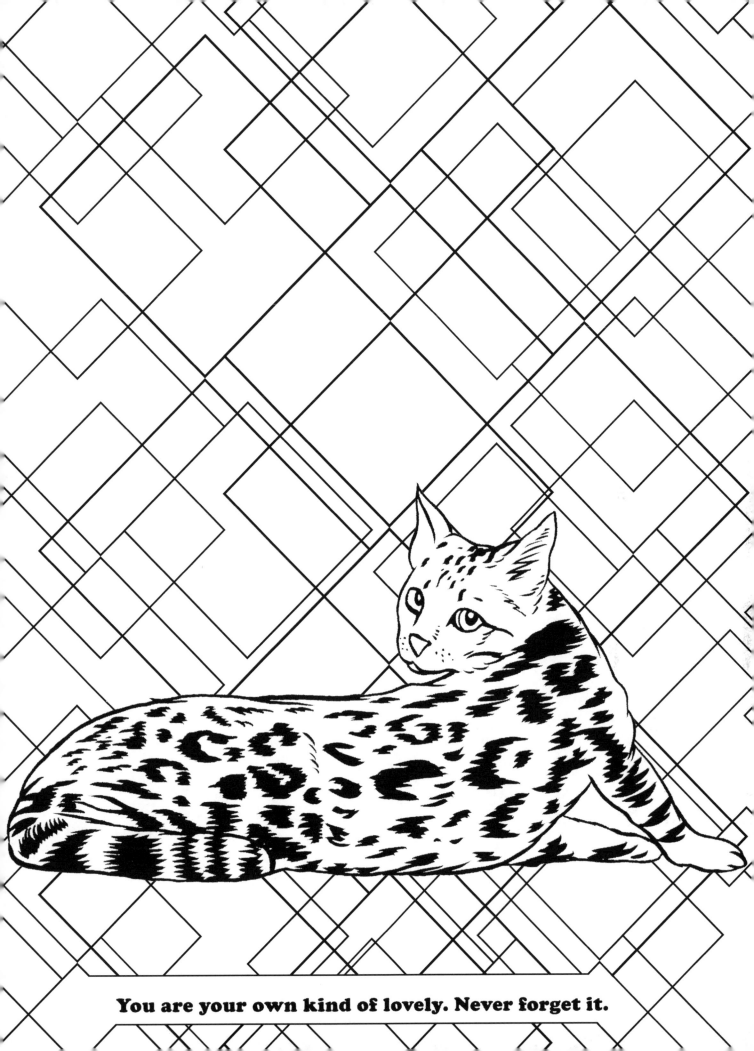

You are your own kind of lovely. Never forget it.

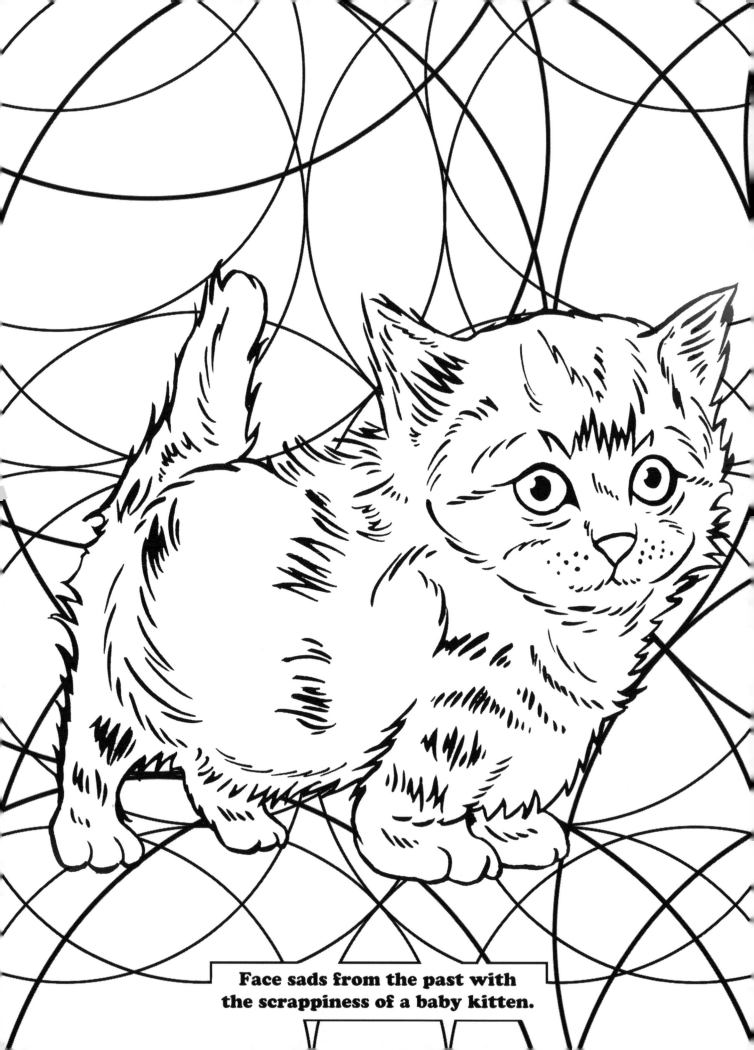

Face sads from the past with
the scrappiness of a baby kitten.

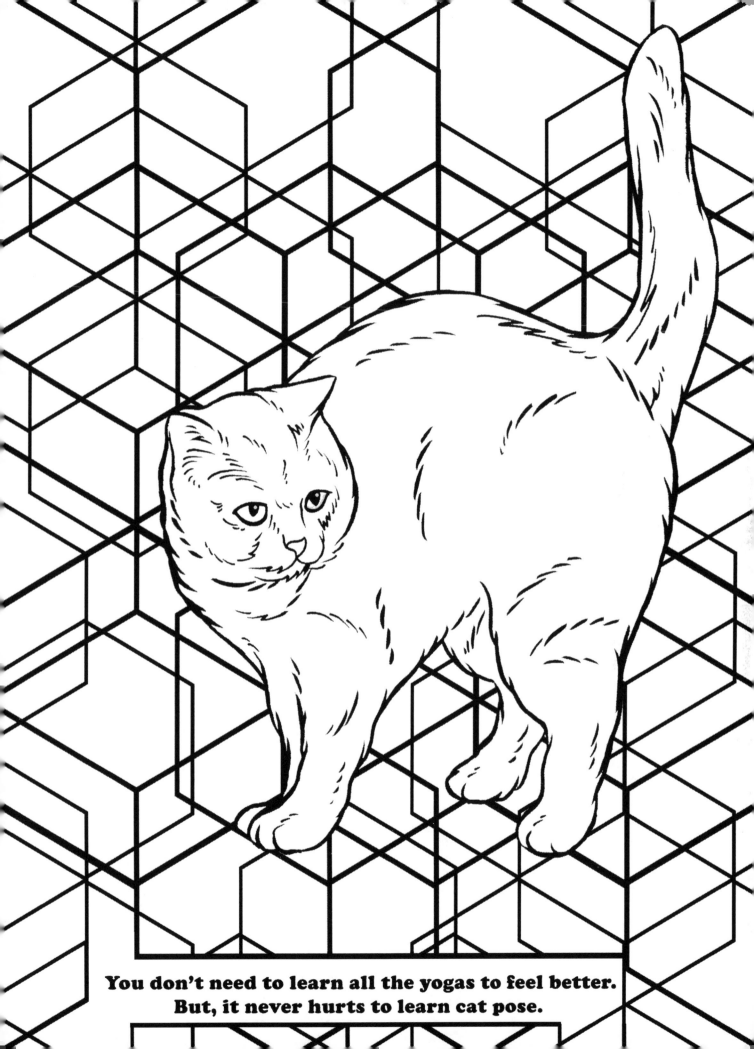

You don't need to learn all the yogas to feel better.
But, it never hurts to learn cat pose.

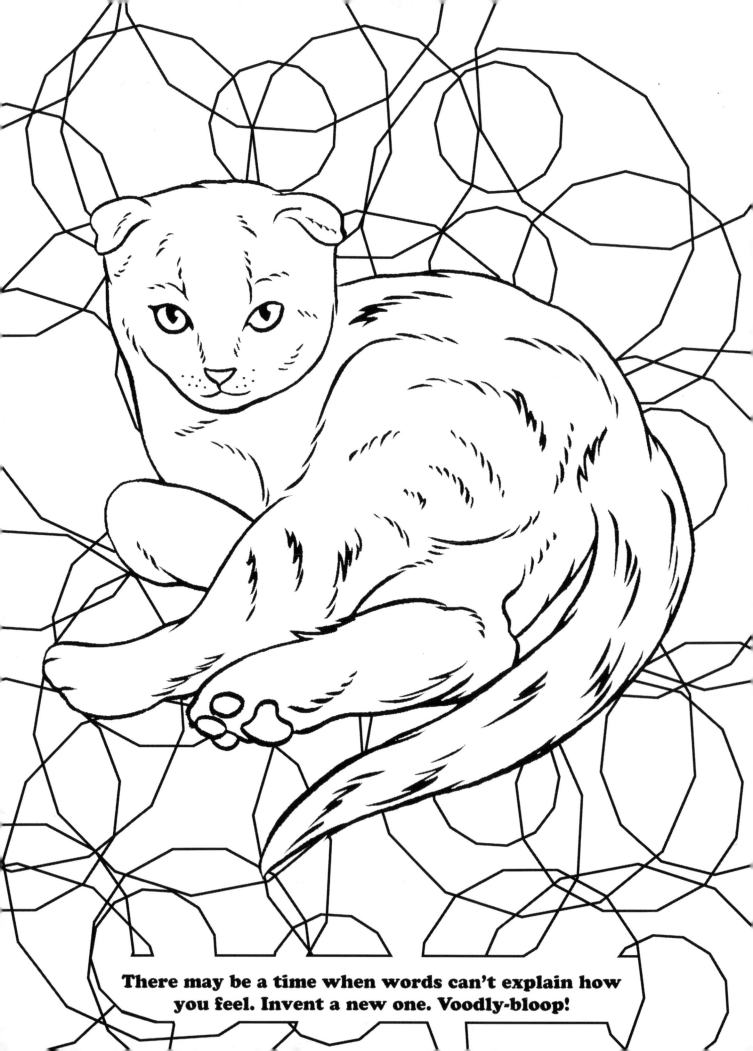

There may be a time when words can't explain how you feel. Invent a new one. Voodly-bloop!

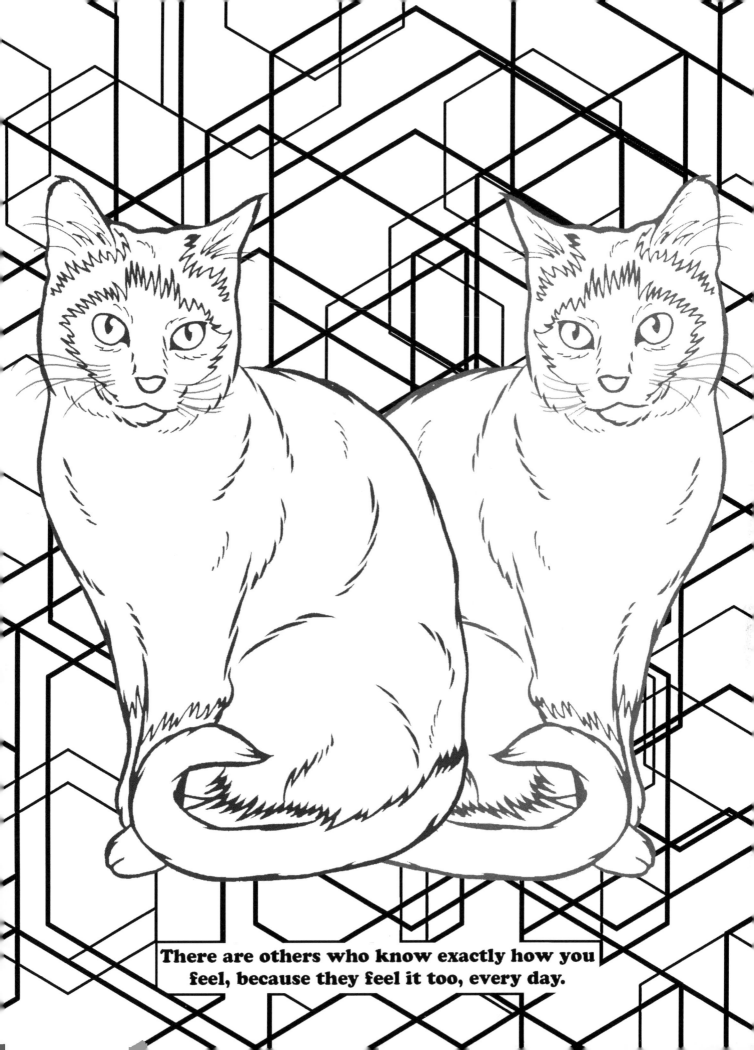

There are others who know exactly how you feel, because they feel it too, every day.

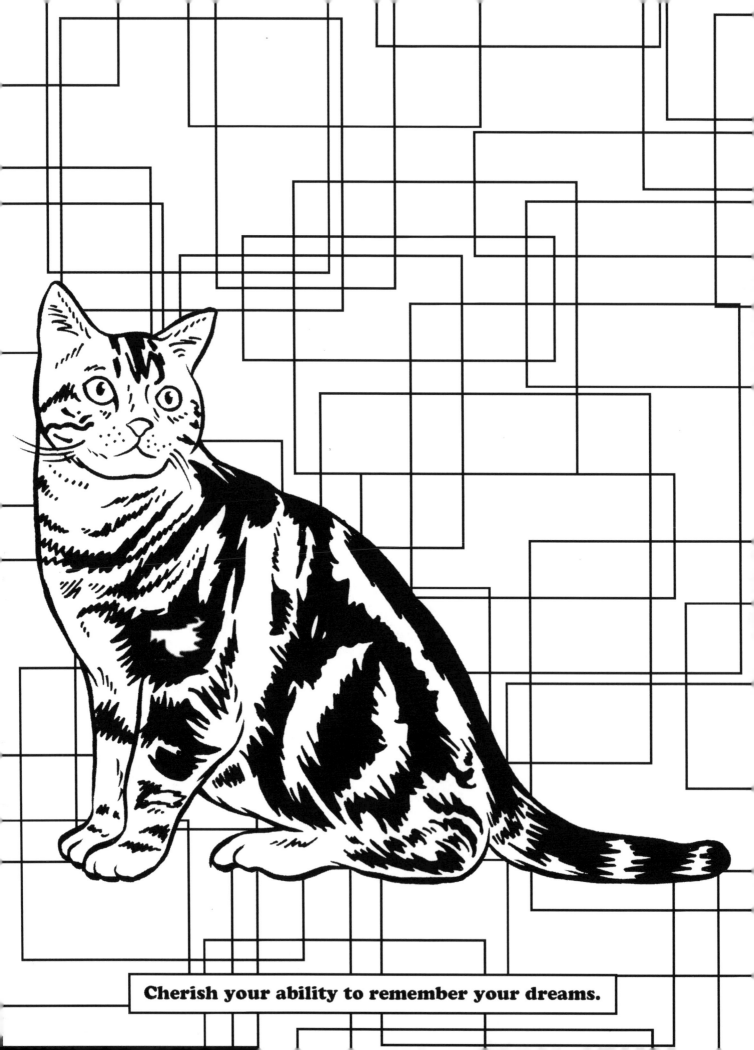

Cherish your ability to remember your dreams.

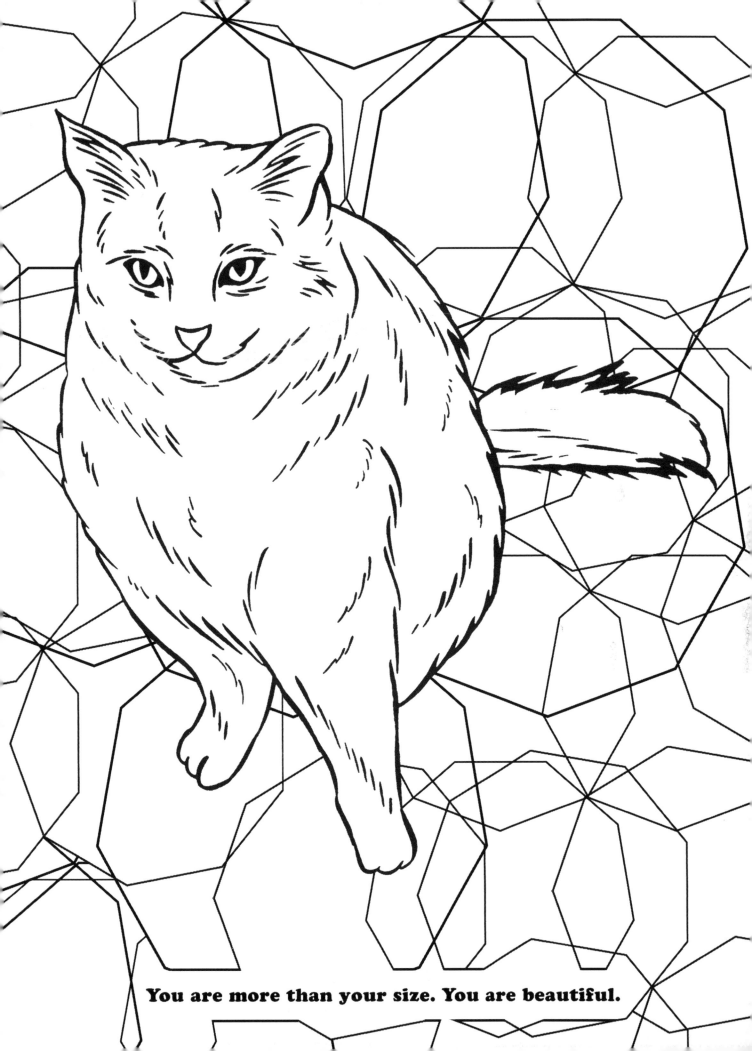

You are more than your size. You are beautiful.

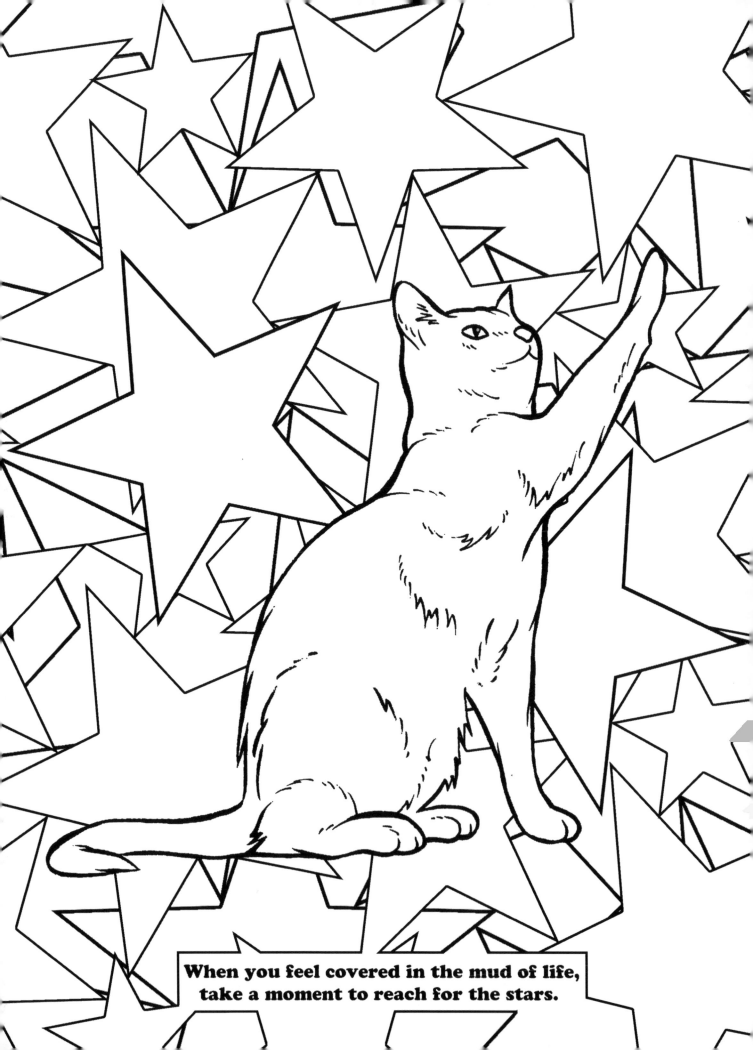

When you feel covered in the mud of life,
take a moment to reach for the stars.

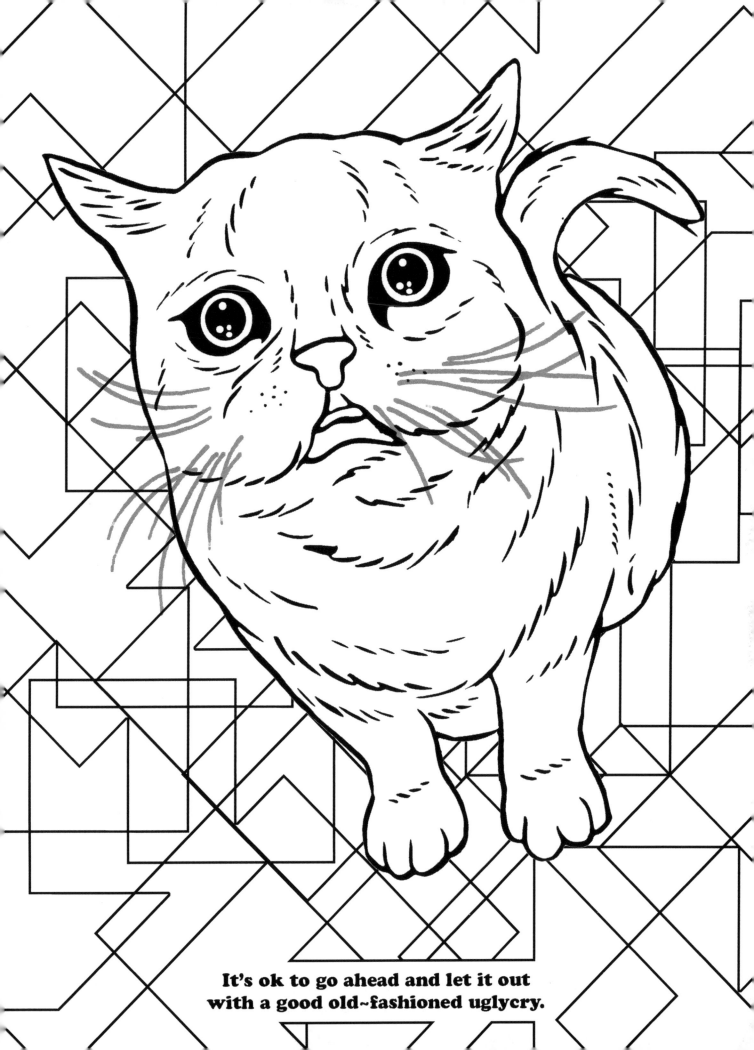

It's ok to go ahead and let it out
with a good old-fashioned uglycry.

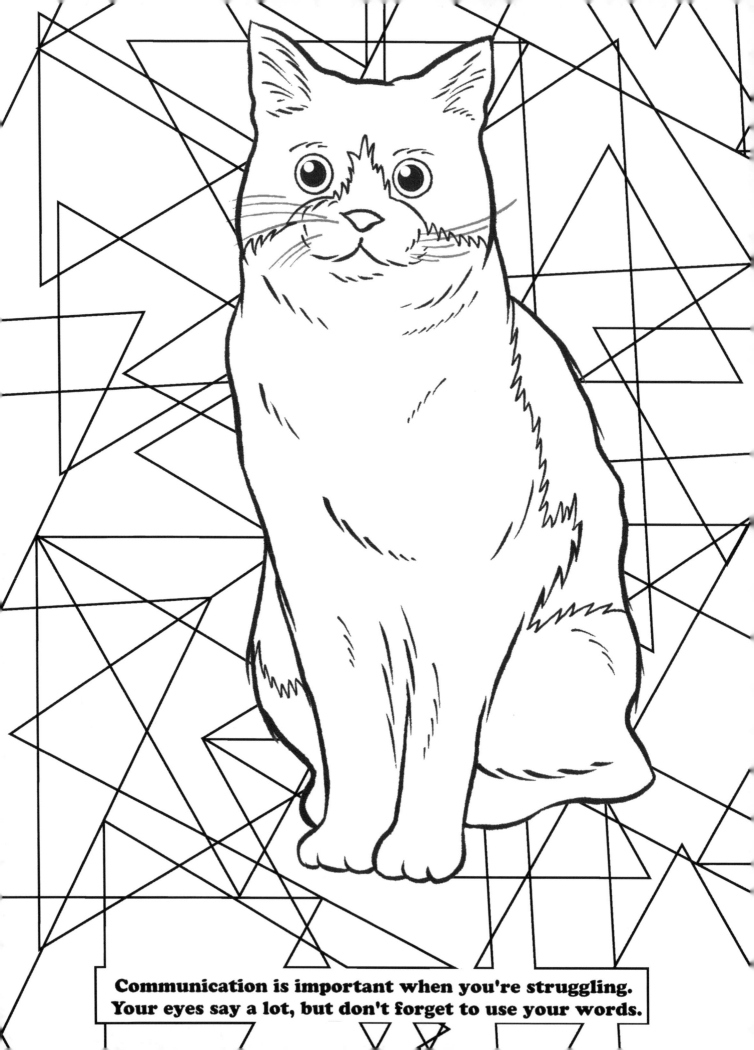

Communication is important when you're struggling.
Your eyes say a lot, but don't forget to use your words.

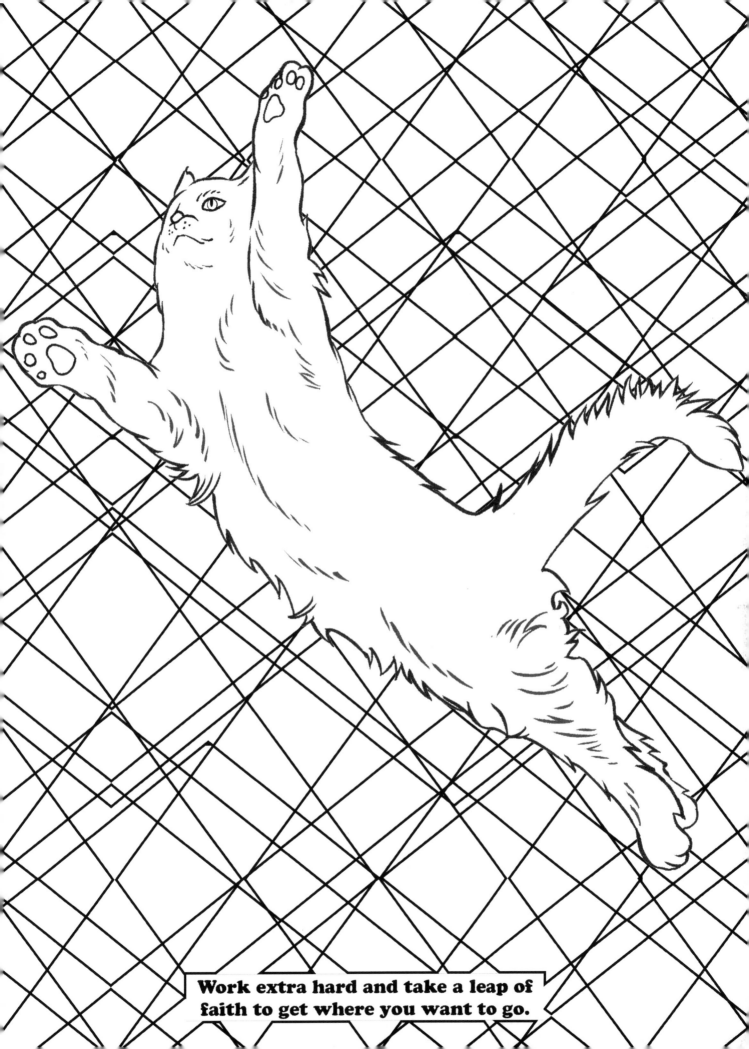

Work extra hard and take a leap of faith to get where you want to go.

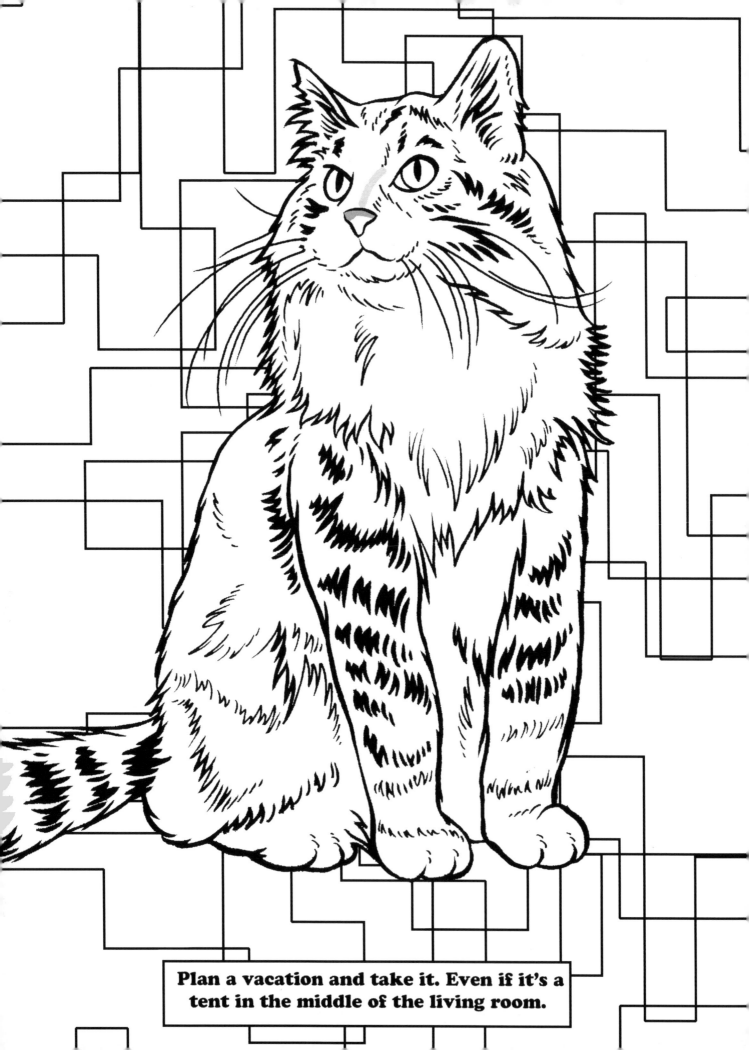

Plan a vacation and take it. Even if it's a tent in the middle of the living room.

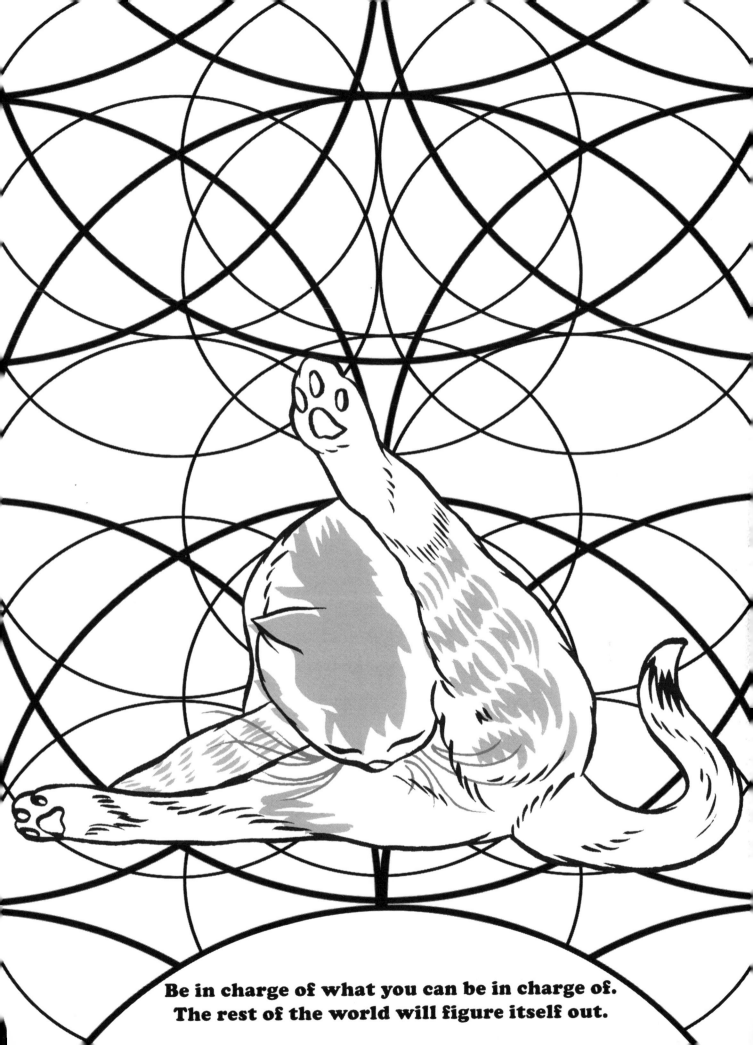

Be in charge of what you can be in charge of.
The rest of the world will figure itself out.

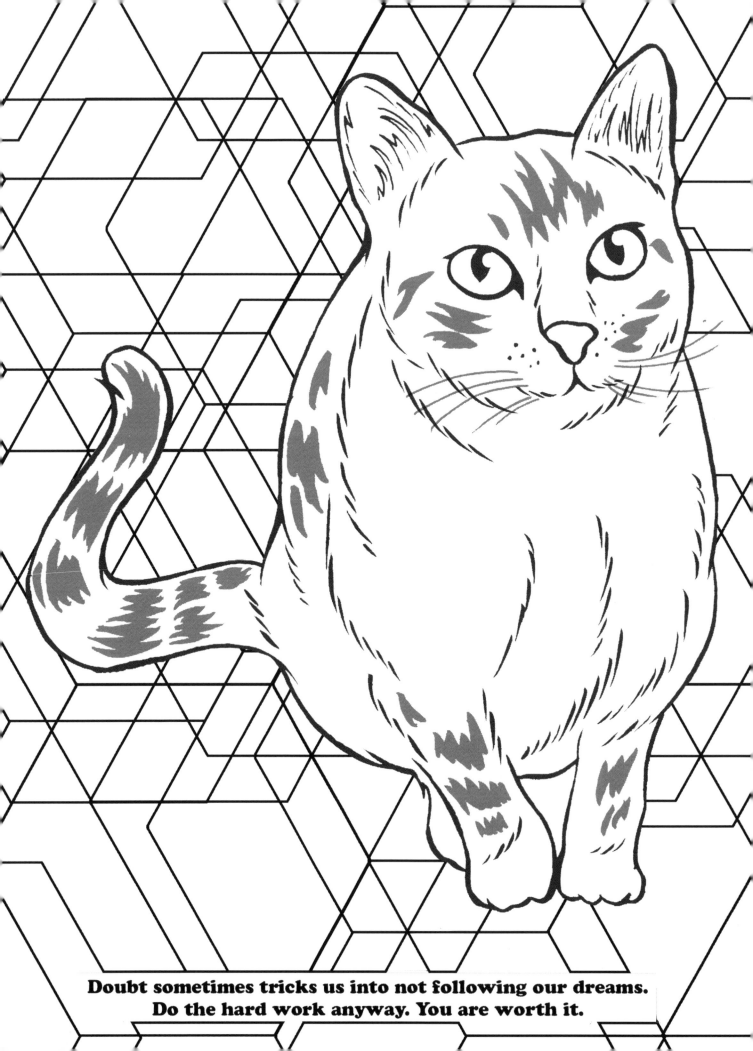

Doubt sometimes tricks us into not following our dreams.
Do the hard work anyway. You are worth it.

Made in the USA
San Bernardino, CA
11 February 2018